GRILLING ......

THE FAMILY

Enjoy Cooking Delicious Smoked

Recipes Outdoors to Share with

Family and Friends + 50 Recipes

By

American Chef's Table

electronic means or in printed format. Recording of this publication is strictly prohibited and any storage of this document is not allowed unless with written permission from the publisher. All rights reserved.

The information herein is offered for informational purposes solely and is universal as so. The presentation of the information is without a contract or any type of guarantee assurance.

The trademarks that are used are without any consent, and the publication of the trademark is without permission or backing by the trademark owner. All trademarks and brands within this book are for clarifying purposes only and are the owned by the owners themselves s, not affiliated with this document.

Table of Contents

Introduction

The moments of family reunions when a barbecue was prepared are unforgettable. Remember those childhood moments when you would anxiously await, soon to be able to eat some of that delicious and steaming meat or simply watching attentively and learning how the adults were in charge of the preparation of the grilled meat. Surely, as you got older, it would be your turn to be in charge of the barbecue.

Although we looked forward to it as children, the task of preparing barbecue is no simple thing, especially if you have to constantly watch the grill and leave the excellent company of family and friends for a while.

The Traeger Grill and Smoker facilitates this scenario, with its functions that allow you to choose the cooking method, temperature and operating time, so you can spend more time with your loved ones.

Since it has automated controls, you can remotely control the fan to feed the fire and the speed at which wood pellets are added to the burn hopper. Don't forget that you will need to be near an electrical outlet to use the pellet grill and that at the end, there will be ashes to clean up.

These are small details to keep in mind, but they will not prevent us from enjoying the best flavor of grilled meats or any type of food that we can prepare like a professional or like a chef and that will amaze those who try it.

Let us not forget that grilled meat is usually accompanied with salads, bread, vegetables and a good red wine. None of this should be missing on the table. The typical salad: tomato, lettuce and onion or any of its varieties. The bread or vegetables can be toasted on the grill and the wine should be served alone, preferably chilled.

You can also grill any of the side dishes, appetizers and desserts presented in this cookbook, with which you can combine flavors, ingredients such as meat, poultry, fish, seafood, all the vegetables you want and various cooking methods such as grilled, barbecued, roasted, baked, to take your culinary skills to a higher level and get the most out of your Trager Grill and Smoker.

Chapter 1: Traeger Grill

Appetizers, Sides & Snacks

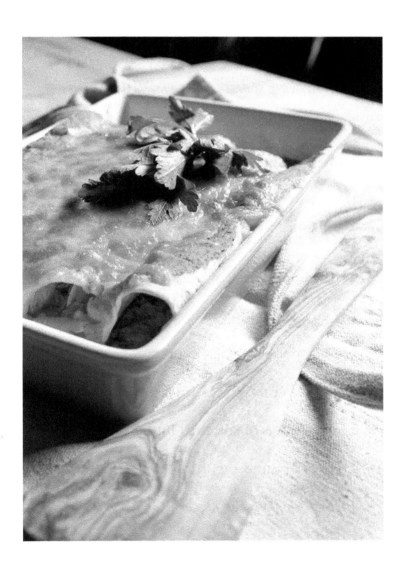

1. Pulled Pork Enchiladas with Smoke-Roasted Red Sauce

(Ready in about: 1 hour & 15 minutes | Serving: 8 | Difficulty: Easy)

Nutrition per serving: Kcal 335 | Fat 15 g | Net Carbs 30 g | Protein 12 g

Ingredients

- 1 small chopped onion

- 1/3 cup of parmesan cheese, grated

- 1/2 cup of shredded cheddar cheese

- 4 russet potatoes, cut into 1/4 inch thick

- 1/2 cup of shredded mozzarella cheese

- 1/2 teaspoon of black pepper

- 1 and 1/2 cups of cream

- 2 tablespoons of softened butter

- 2 cloves of minced garlic

- 2 teaspoons of seasoned salt

- 1 tablespoon of chives

- 1/2 teaspoon of salt

- 2 tablespoons of all-purpose flour

Instructions

1. Let the grill preheat to 375 °F.

2. Oil the 10-inch skillet with cooking spray.

3. In a bowl, add garlic, flour, and 1/2 of cream. Mix well.

4. Add onion and potatoes into the skillet, sprinkle with 1/2 seasoning.

5. Add 1/2 of the sauce over potatoes, add another layer of onion and potato on top. Add 1/2 of the seasoning and sauce over.

6. Bake for 45-50 minutes on a pellet grill. Turn the pan halfway.

7. Mix cheeses in a bowl and add over top of potatoes and bake for 10-15 minutes until cheese is melted and bubbly.

8. Sprinkle the chives and serve.

2. Traeger Grilled Zucchini & Yellow Squash

(Ready in about: 15 minutes | Serving: 8 | Difficulty: Easy)

Nutrition per serving: Kcal 48 | Fat 2 g | Net Carbs 7 g | Protein 2 g

Ingredients

- 2 teaspoons of avocado oil

- 2 zucchinis

- 1 tablespoon of Greek freak seasoning

- 2 yellow squashes

Instructions

1. Let the grill preheat to 375 °F.

2. Cut the squash into quarters, coat with oil, and sprinkle with seasoning.

3. Place on Traeger and cook for 10-15 minutes. After 3-4 minutes, turn the squash.

4. Serve hot.

3. Grilled Mexican Street Corn

(Ready in about: 25 minutes | Serving: 4 | Difficulty: Easy)

Nutrition per serving: Kcal 262 | Fat 20 g | Net Carbs 21 g | Protein 5 g

Ingredients

- 4 corns on the cobb

- 4 tablespoons of mayonnaise

- 2 tablespoons of butter

- 1/4 cup of crumbled Cotija cheese

- 1 teaspoon of salt

- 1/4 cup of chopped cilantro

- Two limes

- 1/2 teaspoon of chili powder

Instructions

1. Coat the cobbs with 1 tablespoon of butter and 1/4 teaspoon of salt.

2. Wrap the coated cobbs with aluminum foil and place them on the grill.

3. Let grill for 20 minutes and turn every 5 minutes. Do not burn the corns.

4. Remove the foil, and spread mayonnaise on cobbs.

5. Add the chili powder, crumbled Cotija cheese, and cilantro.

6. Serve with lime.

4. Smoked Eggs

(Ready in about: 2 hours and 10 minutes | Serving: 12| Difficulty: Easy)

Nutrition per serving: Kcal 189| Fat 7 g| Net Carbs 2 g| Protein 16 g

Ingredients

- 12 eggs

Topping:

- BBQ sauce

Instructions

1. Preheat the Traeger to 325 °F.
2. Put eggs directly on the grill and cook for 1/2 an hour, with the lid closed.
3. Take eggs out and place them in ice water.
4. Lower the grill's temperature to 175 °F.
5. Peel eggs and put again on the grill and cook for 1/2 an hour to 1 hour.
6. Baste eggs with BBQ sauce and serve.

5. Traeger Smoked Baked Potato

(Ready in about: 3 hours and 10 minutes | Serving: 6| Difficulty: Easy)

Nutrition per serving: Kcal 370| Fat 8 g| Net Carbs 64 g| Protein 8 g

Ingredients

- 1 tablespoon of Kosher salt

- 6 russet potatoes

- 1/4 cup of avocado oil

For Toppings:

- Butter

- Sour Cream

- Chives

- Bacon

- Cheddar Cheese

Instructions

1. Let the pellet grill preheat to 200-220 °F.

2. Clean the potatoes and pierce with a fork all over.

3. Put potatoes on the grill at 200 °F for 2 hours.

4. Take the potatoes out and raise the temperature to 400 °F.

5. Coat potatoes with oil and salt.

6. Put the potatoes back on the grill for 1 hour until fork tender.

7. Serve with toppings.

Chapter 2: Traeger Grill Pork

Recipes

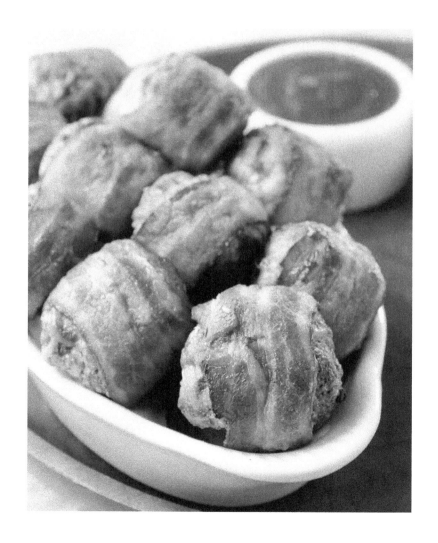

6. Smoked Bacon Wrapped Meatballs

(Ready in about: 2 hours and 10 minutes | Serving: 8 | Difficulty: Medium)

Nutrition per serving: Kcal 243 | Fat 17 g | Net Carbs 13 g | Protein 17.8 g

Ingredients

- 1/2 tablespoon of kosher salt
- 1 pound of Italian sausage
- 1/4 tablespoon of black pepper
- 1 pound of ground beef
- 1 tablespoon of paprika
- 2 jalapenos
- 1 pound of bacon
- 1 cup of cheddar cheese
- 1 whole egg

Instructions

1. Slice the jalapenos, may or may not remove seeds.

2. Cut the bacon in half.

3. In a bowl, mix seasonings, meat, and egg. With clean hands, mix and set it aside.

4. Slice the cheese into 8   portions.

5. Divide the meat into 8   balls and place on parchment paper. Flatten them and add cheese and jalapeno and again shape them into a ball.

6. Wrap the balls in bacon slices, secure with a toothpick.

7. Place meatballs in Trager and cook for 1 hour at 225 °F

8. Raise the heat to 350 °F after 1 hour and cook until the internal temperature reaches 160 °F.

7. Smoked Spicy Asian Pork Ribs

(Ready in about: 6 hours and 15 minutes | Serving: 15 | Difficulty: Medium)

Nutrition per serving: Kcal 612 | Fat 29 g | Net Carbs 38 g | Protein33 g

Ingredients

- 1/2 cup of Togarashi seasoning
- 2 racks of baby back ribs

Sauce:

- 1/4 cup of rice wine vinegar
- 1 cup of soy sauce
- 1 tablespoon of Sriracha
- 2 tablespoons of garlic chili paste
- 1 cup of sweet chili sauce
- 1 teaspoon of powdered ginger
- 1/2 cup of pineapple juice

Instructions

1. Let the grill preheat to 180-190 °F or smoke setting.

2. Coat ribs with Togarashi mix and place on grill.

3. Smoke for 4-5 hours.

4. In a bowl, add all the sauce ingredients, mix well.

5. Put ribs in a pan and pour the sauce all over, cover with foil.

6. Put back on the grill and cook at 250-275 °F for 2-3 hours, but keep checking after every hour.

8. Grilled Bacon-Wrapped Pork Chops with Rosemary

(Ready in about: 1 hour | Serving: 6| Difficulty: Medium)

Nutrition per serving: Kcal 395|Fat 22 g| Net Carbs 2 g| Protein 23 g

Ingredients

- 6 slices of bacon
- 6 pork chops, center-cut
- 6 sprigs rosemary
- 2 tablespoons of Dry BBQ rub

Instructions

1. Let the Traeger preheat to 325 °F. Coat the pork chops dry BBQ rub.
2. Put 1 rosemary sprig on each pork chop, wrap in bacon. Secure with a toothpick.
3. Cook for 10 minutes and turn it over. Cook until the internal temperature shows 145 °F.
4. Remove and serve right away.

9. Traeger Pork Tenderloin with Mustard Sauce

(Ready in about: 25 minutes | Serving: 4 | Difficulty: Medium)

Nutrition per serving: Kcal 87 | Fat 6 g | Net Carbs 2 g | Protein 6 g

Ingredients

- 1 pork tenderloin
- 1 and 1/2 tablespoons of cooking oil
- 1 teaspoon of red pepper flake
- 1 and 1/2 tablespoons of Dijon mustard
- 1 teaspoon of paprika
- 1/2 teaspoon of onion powder
- 3/4 teaspoon of salt
- 1/2 teaspoon of parsley flakes
- 1/2 teaspoon of granulated garlic
- 1 and 1/2 tablespoons of white vinegar
- 1/4 teaspoon of ground black pepper

Instructions

1. Let the pellet grill preheat to 350 °F.

2. Combine all ingredients and rub onto pork well.

3. Put on grill cook for 20 minutes, turn every 5 minutes until internal temperature reaches 150 °F.

10. Garlic Herb Grilled Pork Chops

(Ready in about: 50 minutes | Serving: 4 | Difficulty: Medium)

Nutrition per serving: Kcal 323 | Fat 6 g | Net Carbs 4 g | Protein 11 g

Ingredients

- 1 cup of olive oil
- 1 tablespoon of Italian seasoning
- 6 pork chops, boneless
- 1/2 teaspoon of black pepper
- 2 tablespoons of lemon juice
- 1 teaspoon of salt
- 4 cloves of minced garlic

Instructions

1. In a bowl, mix Italian seasoning, pepper, olive oil, salt, minced garlic, and lemon juice.
2. Mix it well.
3. In a large sealable bag, add pork chops and pour marinade over and keep in the fridge for 1/2 an hour till 2 hours.
4. Let the Traeger preheat to 400 °F.
5. Cook pork chops on the grill for 3 minutes on each side with the lid closed until the internal temperature reaches 145 °F.

11.   Pigs in Blanket

(Ready in about: 25 minutes | Serving: 6 | Difficulty: Medium)

Nutrition per serving: Kcal 267 | Fat 22 g | Net Carbs 7 g | Protein 9 g

Ingredients

- 1 pack of biscuit dough, refrigerated
- 1 package of hotdogs, slice into thirds

Instructions

1. Let the Traeger preheat to 350 °F.
2. wrap the biscuit dough around cut hot dogs. Place on parchment paper.
3. Place the baking sheet on the grill cook for 20-25 minutes with the lid closed.
4. Cook until biscuits turn golden brown.

Chapter 3: Traeger Grill Beef

Recipes

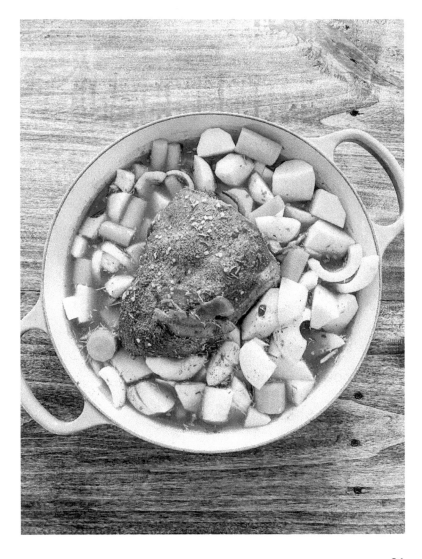

12. Traeger Pot Roast

(Ready in about: 3 hours and 30 minutes | Serving: 8 | Difficulty: Hard)

Nutrition per serving: Kcal 423 | Fat 26 g | Net Carbs 6 g | Protein 39 g

Ingredients

- 2 tablespoons of avocado oil

- 4 cups of beef broth

- 3-4 carrots

- 3-4 pounds of roast beef chuck

- 2 onions

- 1 cup of red wine

- Salt, garlic salt, pepper, seasoned salt, onion powder, as needed

Cornstarch Slurry;

- 1/3 cup of cold water

- 3 tablespoons of cornstarch

Instructions

1. In a cast-iron pan, add oil and place on medium flame.

2. Preheat the Traeger to 275 °F.

3. Season meat with dry spices generously.

4. Brown the meat in cast iron for 4-5 minutes.

5. Add carrots, red wine, sliced onions, broth to pan.

6. Place pan on grill and cook for 2-3 hours.

7. Raise the temperature of Traeger to 325 °F until the internal temperature of beef reaches 200 °F.

8. Take the pan off the grill and take out vegetables and meat and cover with foil.

9. Let the juices in the pan simmer. Add more broth to make it 3 cups.

10. Add cornstarch slurry to the pan. Mix until thickens.

11. Serve roast and vegetables with gravy.

13. Marinated Smoked Flank Steak

(Ready in about: 9 hours and 40 minutes | Serving: 4 | Difficulty: Medium)

Nutrition per serving: Kcal 264 | Fat 9 g | Net Carbs 6 g | Protein 38 g

Ingredients

- 1 teaspoon of garlic powder

- 1 and a half-pound of flank steak

- 1 tablespoon of light brown sugar

- 1 tablespoon of soy sauce

- 1/2 teaspoon of black pepper

- 1 teaspoon of garlic salt

Instructions

1. In a bowl, add all ingredients, except for meat.

2. In a zip lock bag, add meat and marinade ingredients.

3. Mix well and keep in the fridge for 8 hours.

4. Preheat the Traeger to 225 °F. Put the steak on the grill and cook for 1/2 an hour until the internal temperature reaches 135 °F.

5. Serve hot.

14. Mexican Carne Asada

(Ready in about: 5 hours and 15 minutes | Serving: 6 | Difficulty: Medium)

Nutrition per serving: Kcal 519 | Fat 10 g | Net Carbs 62 g | Protein 41 g

Ingredients

- 1 orange juice

- 1/4 cup of Worcestershire sauce

- 2 pounds of flank steak, thinly cut

- 2 tablespoons of white wine vinegar

- Salt and cumin to taste

- 4 garlic cloves

- 1/4 of an onion

- 2 tablespoons of black pepper

Instructions

1. In a zip lock bag, add all ingredients of the marinade and mix well. Add in steak.

2. Keep in the fridge for 5 hours. Do not over marinate.

3. Preheat the Traeger to 375 °F.

4. Cook the steak directly on the grill. Flipping, so it does not become dry.

5. Serve in tortillas.

15. Baked Corned Beef Au Gratin

(Ready in about: 1 hour | Serving: 6| Difficulty: Medium)

Nutrition per serving: Kcal 289 | Fat 12 g| Net Carbs 14 g| Protein 21 g

Ingredients

- 1 pound of corned beef

- 2 tablespoons of butter, softened

- 1/2 cup of whole milk

- 2 tablespoons of all-purpose flour

- 4 cloves of minced garlic

- 3 pounds of russet potatoes

- 1 and 1/2 cups of heavy cream

- 1 teaspoon of kosher salt

- 1 sliced onion

- Black pepper, to taste

Instructions

1. Preheat the Traeger to 450 °F.

2. Take a 9" cast iron pan, coat with butter. In a bowl, add minced garlic, cream, salt, black pepper, flour, and milk mix.

3. In the skillet, add onions, corned beef, and 1/3 of potatoes. Pour 1/3 cream mixture over potatoes.

4. Keep layering until all cream mix is used.

5. Bake for 1/2 an hour on the grill, cover with aluminum foil.

6. Take off foil and bake for 20 more minutes, until potatoes are brownish.

7. Add shredded cheese on top and bake for 3-5 minutes.

8. Serve.

16. Traeger Smoked Meatloaf

(Ready in about: 1 hour and 5 minutes | Serving: 12 | Difficulty: Medium)

Nutrition per serving: Kcal 198 | Fat 5 g | Net Carbs 32 g | Protein 19 g

Ingredients

Meatloaf:

- 3 pounds ground beef
- 1 diced onion
- 2 egg yolks
- 1/4 cup of milk
- 3 whole eggs
- 1/2 cup of Ketchup
- 1/2 cup of panko breadcrumbs
- 1/2 teaspoon of salt
- 1/2 teaspoon of dry mustard
- 1/4 teaspoon of black pepper
- 1/4 teaspoon of garlic powder

- 1 teaspoon of dried parsley

- 1/2 teaspoon of onion powder

- 2 cups of saltine crackers, crushed

- 1 tablespoon of minced garlic

For Sauce:

- 1 and 1/2 cup of light brown sugar

- 1 and 1/2 cups of apple cider vinegar

- 1/4 cup of Ketchup

- 1 tablespoon of yellow mustard

Instructions

1. Preheat the Traeger to 325 °F.

2. In a pan, mix all ingredients of the sauce. Let it simmer until it reduces and thickens.

3. In a bowl, add all other ingredients except for beef. Mix well, then add ground beef. Do not over mix.

4. In a foil pan, press the beef mixture. Leave some space between the pan and loaf.

5. Pour 1/3 of the sauce over.

6. Place on grill and cook for 1/2 an hour or until it sets and completely cooked.

7. Flip onto grill and brush with glaze cook with lid closed for 10 minutes. Baste with sauce again cook for 10 to 15 minutes until internal temperature reaches 160 °F.

8. Take off the grill, rest, and serve.

17. Traeger Smoked Mississippi Pot Roast

(Ready in about: 5 hours and 15 minutes | Serving: 8| Difficulty: Medium)

Nutrition per serving: Kcal 314| Fat 13 g| Net Carbs 4 g| Protein 39 g

Ingredients

- 1 stick of salted butter

- 5 pounds of beef roast chuck

- 1 teaspoon of black pepper

- 1 teaspoon of paprika

- 1 teaspoon of onion powder

- 8 pepperoncini peppers

- 1/4 cup of carrots, chopped

- 1 packet of au jus mix

- 1 teaspoon of salt

- 1/2 teaspoon of granulated garlic

- 1 packet of dressing dry ranch mix

- 1/2 a cup of water

Instructions

1. Coat the roast with all dry spices.

2. Sear the roast in cast iron on each side.

3. Preheat the Traeger grill to 275 °F.

4. In a large grill-safe pan, add seared meat with butter, ranch mix, pepperoncini, water, carrots, jus, and garlic. Place this pan on the grill and close the lid.

5. Let it cook and monitor so it would not burn after every hour.

6. Cook until it becomes fork tender or internal temperature reaches 200-205 °F.

7. Serve with bread and mashed potatoes.

18. Brisket Chili

(Ready in about: 60 minutes | Serving: 12 | Difficulty: Medium)

Nutrition per serving: Kcal 385 | Fat 8 g | Net Carbs 17 g | Protein 31 g

Ingredients

- 15 ounces of tomato sauce

- 4 cups of cooked brisket, diced

- 1 can of chili beans

- 2 cans of stewed tomatoes

- 8 cups of water

- Sour cream, to your taste

- 1 package of chili kit

- 1 can drain of pinto beans

- Cheese, as needed

Instructions

1. In a pot, add all ingredients except for beans.

2. Let it simmer on low heat for 45 minutes. Add in beans.

3. Preheat the Traeger to 375 °F.

4. Place the pot on the grill and cook for 1/2 an hour.

5. Serve with cheese and sour cream.

Chapter 4: Traeger Grill

Poultry Recipes

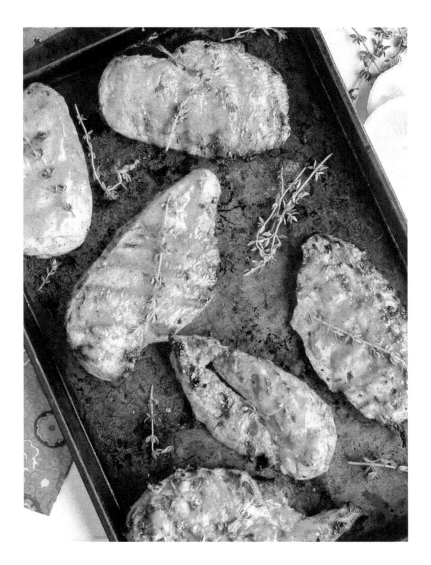

19. Savory Grilled Chicken

(Ready in about: 1 hour | Serving: 6| Difficulty: Medium)

Nutrition per serving: Kcal 378 | Fat 28 g| Net Carbs 2 g| Protein 38 g

Ingredients

- 2 and 1/2 pounds of skinless, boneless chicken breasts
- 1 tablespoon of Worcestershire sauce
- 1/4 cup of white wine vinegar
- Juice from 1/2 lemon
- 3 tablespoons of mayonnaise
- 1/2 cup of olive oil
- 2 teaspoons of fresh thyme
- 1 teaspoon of smoked paprika
- 1 teaspoon of salt and black pepper, each
- 1/2 tablespoons of onion powder
- 1 clove of minced garlic

Instructions

1. In a bowl, add all ingredients except for chicken, mix well.

2. In a large zip lock bag, pour marinade and chicken. Coat the chicken well.

3. Marinade for 1/2 an hour or a whole day

4. Let the grill preheat to 400-500 °F

5. Grill the chicken until cooked through or for 5 minutes on each side.

20. Greek Chicken Marinade

(Ready in about: 1 hour and 5 minutes | Serving: 2 | Difficulty: Medium)

Nutrition per serving: Kcal 313 | Fat 24 g | Net Carbs 6.8 g | Protein 35 g

Ingredients

- 3 pounds of chicken thighs or drumsticks

- 1 and 1/2 cups plain yogurt

- 2 teaspoons of salt

- 1/2 cup of olive oil

- 1 teaspoon of black pepper

- 1 teaspoon of fresh chopped thyme

- 1 teaspoon of lemon zest

- 1/3 cup of fresh lemon juice

- 2 teaspoons of fresh chopped dill

- 8 cloves of minced garlic

- 1 teaspoon of fresh chopped rosemary

- 1 teaspoon of oregano

Instructions

1. In a bowl, add lemon juice, yogurt, garlic, pepper, herbs, salt, and olive oil. Mix well

2. Add in chicken and coat well; keep in the fridge for 2 hours or all night.

3. Preheat Traeger to 400 °F.

4. Place chicken on a baking sheet and place the sheet on grill cook for until internal temperature reaches 170 °F

5. Serve hot.

21. Easy Grilled Curry Chicken

(Ready in about: 30 minutes | Serving: 2 | Difficulty: Medium)

Nutrition per serving: Kcal 336 | Fat 21 g | Net Carbs 7 g | Protein 37 g

Ingredients

- 2 teaspoons of smoked paprika

- 2 teaspoons of curry powder

- 2 tablespoons of apple sauce

- 1/2 teaspoon of salt

- 3 tablespoons of coconut milk

- 2 tablespoons of corn oil

- 1/2 teaspoon of turmeric powder

- Two chicken breasts

- 1 teaspoon of black pepper

Instructions

1. In a bowl, add turmeric, pepper, smoked paprika, curry powder, oil, salt, and corn oil, mix well.

2. Add in coconut milk, apple sauce to make a paste.

3. Coat the chicken well with this paste.

4. Preheat the Traeger to 375 °F.

5. Cook chicken directly on the grill for 5 to 8 minutes until the thermometer reaches 165 °F.

6. Serve hot.

7.39 Gold BBQ Grilled Chicken

(Ready in about: 4 hour and 26 minutes | Serving: 4 | Difficulty: Easy)

Nutrition per serving: Kcal 276 | Fat 9 g | Net Carbs 15 g | Protein 32 g

Ingredients

- 1-1.5 skinless, boneless chicken breasts
- Grilling & Finishing sauce of Carolina Gold

Marinade:

- 1/4 cup of apple cider vinegar
- 1/4 cup of olive oil
- 1 teaspoon of lemon juice
- 1 teaspoon of sugar
- 1/4 teaspoon of white pepper
- 1 teaspoon of Worcestershire sauce
- 2 cloves of minced garlic
- 1 teaspoon of onion powder
- 1 teaspoon of kosher salt

Instructions

1. In a large sealable, add all the marinade ingredients, add chicken mix, and keep in the fridge for 4 hours.

2. Preheat the Traeger to 375 °F.

3. Take chicken out and pound it so equal thickness.

4. Place pieces directly on the grill.

5. Cook for 6 to 8 minutes on each side, until cooked through or until internal temperature reaches 165 °F.

6. In the last 3 minutes of cooking, brush gold sauce over chicken.

7. Let it rest before serving.

22. Smoked Buttermilk Fried Chicken

(Ready in about: 2 hour and 45 minutes+ brine 12 hours| Serving: 8| Difficulty: Medium)

Nutrition per serving: Kcal 418 | Fat 16 g| Net Carbs 19 g| Protein 46 g

Ingredients

Buttermilk Brine

- 4 pounds of chicken pieces

- 1/2 teaspoon of ground pepper

- 1/2 teaspoon granulated garlic

- 1/4 cup of hot sauce

- 2 cups of buttermilk

- 1/2 teaspoon of salt

Breading

- 1 teaspoon of salt

- black pepper: 1/2 teaspoon

- 2 cups of all-purpose flour

- 1 teaspoon of paprika

- 1 teaspoon mustard powder

- 1 teaspoon baking soda

- 1 teaspoon onion powder

- 1/2 teaspoon cayenne pepper

- 1/2 teaspoon granulated garlic

- 1 teaspoon baking powder

- 1/2 teaspoon of ground thyme

Egg Wash:

- 1/4 cup of whole milk

- 4 whole eggs

Instructions

1. In a large pot, add all ingredients of buttermilk brine, mix well and keep chicken inside. Keep in the fridge overnight.

2. Set the Traeger to smoke or 180 °F. Smoke the brined chicken for 2 hours.

3. Take off from the grill and keep in the fridge to cool completely.

4. Meanwhile, prepare the egg wash, and combine all the ingredients of breading.

5. In a skillet, add 4 to 5 cups of oil keep to 350 °F on the grill. Keep monitoring the temperature of oil using a thermometer.

6. Coat the chicken in the flour mix — place in a rack.

7. Fry chicken pieces a few at a time until crispy.

8. Cook until the internal temperature reaches 165 °F.

9. Serve hot.

23. Pellet Grill Jerk Chicken Thighs

(Ready in about: 1 hour and 20 minutes | Serving: 6 | Difficulty: Easy)

Nutrition per serving: Kcal 619 | Fat 44 g | Net Carbs 7 g | Protein 32 g

Ingredients

- 6 chicken skin-on thighs

- 1/2 teaspoon of cinnamon

- 4 cloves of garlic

- 3 tablespoons of olive oil

- Jerk chicken marinade

- 4 teaspoon salt

- 1 and 1/2 teaspoons of black pepper

- 2 tablespoons of soy sauce

- 1/2 teaspoon of ground nutmeg

- 2 teaspoon of fresh thyme leaves

- 4-5 habanero peppers

- 1 teaspoon of ground allspice

- 1/4 cup of fresh lime juice

- 1 onion

- 1 tablespoon of chopped green onion

- 1 tablespoon of brown sugar

Instructions

1. In a blender, add all ingredients except for chicken, pulse to combine.

2. In a large sealable bag, add marinade and chicken coat well and keep in the fridge overnight.

3. Let the grill preheat to 375 °F. Place chicken on grill skin side down.

4. Cook chicken for 20-25 minutes, flip and grill more until internal temperature shows 165 °F.

5. In a large pan, add 1/2 a cup of oil on medium flame, take the chicken out from the grill.

6. Fry in hot oil to crisp up skin for 2-3 minutes.

7. Serve hot.

24.   Beer Can Chicken

(Ready in about: 1 hour and 40 minutes | Serving: 6 | Difficulty: Easy)

Nutrition per serving: Kcal 718 | Fat 44 g | Net Carbs 8 g | Protein 37 g

Ingredients

- 1/2 cup of chicken rub, dry

- 1 4-5-pound chicken

- 1 can of beer

Instructions

1. Let the grill set to smoke for 4 -5 minutes; keep the lid open. Keep the temperature to high until it reaches 450 °F.

2. Rub chicken with dry rub generously.

3. Keep the chicken whole and add 1/2 beer of can inside the chicken.

4. Cook until the internal temperature reaches 165 °F.

5. Slice and serve.

25. Traeger Chicken Wings with Spicy Miso

(Ready in about: 40 minutes | Serving: 6 | Difficulty: Easy)

Nutrition per serving: Kcal 608 | Fat 34 g | Net Carbs 24 g | Protein 27 g

Ingredients

- 2 pounds of chicken wings

- 1/8 cup of gochujang

- 3/4 cup of soy sauce

- 1 tablespoon of Sriracha

- Togarashi

- 1/8 cup of miso

- 1/2 cup of oil

- 1/2 cup of pineapple juice

- 1/2 cup of water

Instructions

1. In a bowl, add all ingredients, mix well and coat the wings well.

2. Keep in the refrigerator for 8-12 hours.

3. Let the grill preheat to 375 °F.

4. Place wings directly on Traeger, with the lid closed.

5. Grill until the internal temperature reaches 165 °F, or for 25 minutes.

6. Before serving, sprinkle with Togarashi.

Chapter 5: Traeger Grill

Seafood Recipes

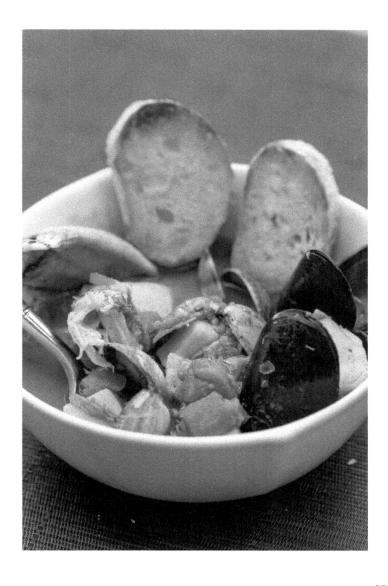

26. Traeger Cioppino

(Ready in about: 1 hour and 5 minutes | Serving: 8 | Difficulty: Medium)

Nutrition per serving: Kcal 711 | Fat 26 g | Net Carbs 22 g | Protein 76 g

Ingredients

Soup Base:

- 6 cups of fish stock

- 1 sliced fennel bulb

- 1/4 cup of butter

- 1 diced carrot

- 4 diced shallots

- 1 diced onion

- 5 cloves of minced garlic

- 2 teaspoons of dried oregano

- 3 sprigs of fresh thyme

- 2 15-ounce cans of diced tomatoes with juices

- 2 cups of dry white

- 1 6-ounce can of tomato paste

- 2 bay leaves

- 1 tablespoon of salt

- 1 teaspoon of red pepper flakes

Seafood:

- 2 pounds of skinless fresh fish, cut into one-inch pieces

- 2 crabs, halved & steamed

- 1 pound of prawns

- 1 pound of cleaned mussels

- 1 pound of cleaned steamer clams

Instructions

1. Preheat the Traeger to 375 °F.

2. In a Dutch oven, add butter on medium flame. Add in diced carrot, a sliced fennel bulb, shallots, and diced onion.

3. Sauté for 2 to 3 minutes, till the vegetables softened.

4. Add garlic and sauté for 30 seconds.

5. Add tomatoes with juice, herbs, fish stock, seasonings, and tomato paste. Let it simmer.

6. Place Dutch oven on the grill, let it simmer for 15 minutes until the stew's internal temperature reaches 180 to 211 °F.

7. Add all seafood.

8. Cook for 10 minutes.

9. Serve hot.

27. Blackened Catfish Tacos

(Ready in about: 25 minutes | Serving: 5 | Difficulty: Medium)

Nutrition per serving: Kcal 515 | Fat 27 g | Net Carbs 21 g | Protein 46 g

Ingredients

- All-purpose rub

- 1 pound of catfish:

- 1 cup of shredded cabbage

- 5 tortillas

- Lemon cut into wedges

- 1 cup of shredded cheese

Tartar Sauce

- 1 cup of mayo

- 1 diced cucumber

- 3 tablespoons of wasabi paste

- Juice from 2 lemons

- 1 brick of cream cheese

- 1 diced onion

- 1/4 cup of dill pickle relish

Instructions

1. Coat the fish in seasoning rub. Keep in the fridge.

2. In a bowl, add onion, cream cheese, mayo, and mix well.

3. Add in wasabi paste, 1/4 cup of dill pickle relish, cucumber, lemon juice of 1 lemon, salt, and pepper. Mix well. Keep in the fridge.

4. Preheat the Traeger to 350 °F., and place the fish on grill grates. Cook on one side for 10 minutes.

5. Take off grill and serve in tacos with tartar sauce, cabbage and. cheese

28. Traeger Honey Garlic Salmon

(Ready in about: 25 minutes | Serving: 6| Difficulty: Medium)

Nutrition per serving: Kcal 619| Fat 36 g| Net Carbs 17 g| Protein 49 g

Ingredients

Sauce:

- 3 tablespoons of butter

- 3 tablespoons of soy sauce

- 1/3 cup of honey

- 2 tablespoons of white wine

- 2 tablespoons of minced garlic

- 3 tablespoons of balsamic vinegar

Salmon:

- Olive oil

- 6 small salmon filets

- Garlic powder

- Salt and pepper

- Onion powder

Instructions

1. Preheat the Traeger to 350 °F

2. In a bowl, add all ingredients of the sauce.

3. Pour this mix into a grill-safe dish

4. Coat salmon with olive oil and sprinkle with seasoning; place salmon in foil pan.

5. Place both pans on the grill and cook for 10-20 minutes or until salmon's internal temperature reaches 145 °F.

6. Cook the sauce for 10   minutes. Do not burn.

7. Take both pans out of the grill.

8. Pour sauce over salmon and serve.

29.   Traeger Lobster Rolls

(Ready in about: 15 minutes | Serving: 4 | Difficulty: Easy)

Nutrition per serving: Kcal 234 | Fat 16 g | Net Carbs 16 g | Protein 8 g

Ingredients

- 4 rolls

- 4 lobster tails, grilled but cooled down

- 2 tablespoons of lemon juice

- 1 teaspoon of kosher salt

- 2 tablespoons of chopped parsley

- 1 tablespoon of chopped green onion

- 1 stalk of celery stalk, chopped

- 1/4 cup of mayo

- 1/2 teaspoon of ground black pepper

Instructions

1. In a bowl, add parsley, lemon juice, mayo, green onions, salt, celery, and black pepper mix well. Let it rest for 5-10 minutes.

2. Remove shells from lobster and cut into small pieces

3. Slowly mix the sauce and lobster and the sauce.

4. Toast the buttered buns in a pan. Place lobster and mixture on top.

5. Smoke in Traeger for 10 minutes at 250 °F until heated through.

6. Serve right away.

30. Traeger Tuna Melt Flatbread

(Ready in about: 20 minutes | Serving: 6 | Difficulty: Easy)

Nutrition per serving: Kcal 321 | Fat 15 g | Net Carbs 12 g | Protein 23 g

Ingredients

- 6 flatbreads

- 2 cans of water-packed tuna

- 1/4 teaspoon of garlic powder

- 1/2 teaspoon of salt

- 1/4 teaspoon of onion powder

- 1/2 cup of mayo

- Microgreens

- 3 tablespoons of chopped dill pickles

- 1/4 teaspoon of pepper

- 2 cups of shredded cheese

Instructions

1. Mix all ingredients.

2. Let the Traeger preheat to smoke (180 °F).

3. Place on 6 flatbreads and smoke for 10 minutes in Trager

4. Put microgreens on top

5. Serve and enjoy.

31. Traeger Chimichurri Shrimp

(Ready in about: 18 minutes | Serving: 6 | Difficulty: Easy)

Nutrition per serving: Kcal 388 | Fat 17 g | Net Carbs 4 g | Protein 52 g

Ingredients

- 3 tablespoons of avocado oil
- 3 tablespoons of chimichurri seasoning blend
- 3 pounds of peeled shrimp, deveined

Instructions

1. Preheat the Traeger to 375 F.
2. Thread shrimps on skewers and drizzle oil.
3. Season with chimichurri spice rub.
4. Put on the grill and cook on each side for 2-3 minutes, until cooked.
5. Serve right away

Chapter 6: Traeger Grill Lamb

Recipes

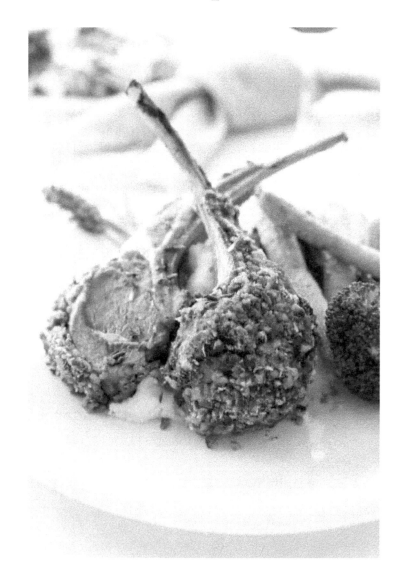

32. Pistachio Crusted Roasted Lamb

(Ready in about: 60 minutes | Serving: 6 | Difficulty: Medium)

Nutrition per serving: Kcal 278 | Fat 13 g | Net Carbs 15 g | Protein 26 g

Ingredients

- 2 racks of lamb
- 1 teaspoon herbs de Provence
- 1 bunch of different color carrots, chopped
- 1 clove of minced garlic
- 1 pound of fingerling potatoes
- 2 tablespoons of vegetable oil
- 3 tablespoons of Dijon mustard
- 2 tablespoons of olive oil
- 2 tablespoons of breadcrumbs
- Salt and black pepper, to taste
- 2 teaspoons of thyme minced
- 2/3 cup of pistachios, chopped

- 1 tablespoon of butter

Instructions

1. Set the Traeger to high, keep the lid closed for 15 minutes.

2. Add 1 tablespoon of vegetable oil to an iron skillet and place on grill. Preheat for 20 minutes with lid closed.

3. Season the lamb rack with salt, herbs de Provence, and pepper.

4. In a bowl, add chopped carrots, olive oil, thyme, salt, potatoes, garlic, and black pepper. Mix well.

5. Put the lamb in a skillet, brown on every side, cook for 6-8 minutes. Take out the Lamb in a baking pan.

6. In a bowl, mix olive oil, salt, pepper, bread crumbs, pistachios, and butter.

7. Spread mustard on the rack of lamb and coat with pistachio mixture.

8. Place coated lamb on the grill directly. Add seasoned carrots and potatoes in the previous skillet on the grill.

9. Keep the lid close, cook for 15 minutes.

10. Stir vegetables after 15 minutes, cover the lamb with foil.

11. Cook for 5-10 minutes more, until the internal temperature of the meat reaches 125 °F.

12. Let the lamb rest on the grill. Take out vegetables if tender.

13. Serve the lamb with roasted vegetables.

33. Rosemary Lamb

(Ready in about: 3 hours | Serving: 6 | Difficulty: Easy)

Nutrition per serving: Kcal 266 | Fat 9.9 g | Net Carbs 6 g | Protein 22 g

Ingredients

- 1 bunch of asparagus

- 2 tablespoons of olive oil

- 1/2 cup of butter

- Black pepper

- Salt, to taste

- 1 dozen baby potato

- 1 rack of lamb ribs

- 2 rosemary springs

Instructions

1. Preheat the Traeger to 225 °F.

2. Trim the membrane of ribs and coat with olive oil and rosemary

3. In a baking dish, mix butter with potatoes.

4. Place ribs on the grill with potatoes.

5. Smoke until internal temperature reaches 145 °F or for 3 hours.

6. In the last 20 minutes of cooking, add asparagus to potatoes until tender.

7. Serve the lamb with vegetables.

34. Chipotle Lamb

(Ready in about: 2 hours | Serving: 6 | Difficulty: Easy)

Nutrition per serving: Kcal 256 | Fat 9.2 g | Net Carbs 9 g | Protein 24 g

Ingredients

- 3/4 cup of olive oil

- 2 tablespoons fresh thyme

- 2 tablespoons Italian parsley

- 1 tablespoon chipotle peppers crushed

- 1 rack of lamb ribs

- Black pepper

- 1/4 cup bacon rub

- 2 tablespoons fresh rosemary

- 3 cloves of garlic

- 2 tablespoons fresh sage

Instructions

1. Let the Traeger preheat to 275 °F.

2. In a bowl, add thyme, rosemary, Italian parsley, oregano, cilantro, ¼ cup olive oil, sage, 1/4 bacon rub, garlic cloves.

3. Spread the rub on lamb ribs.

4. Smoke ribs until internal temperature reach 120-125 °F.

5. Raise the temperature to 425 °F and cook until 135-145 °F.

6. Let it rest before serving.

Chapter 7: Traeger Grill

Vegetables Recipes

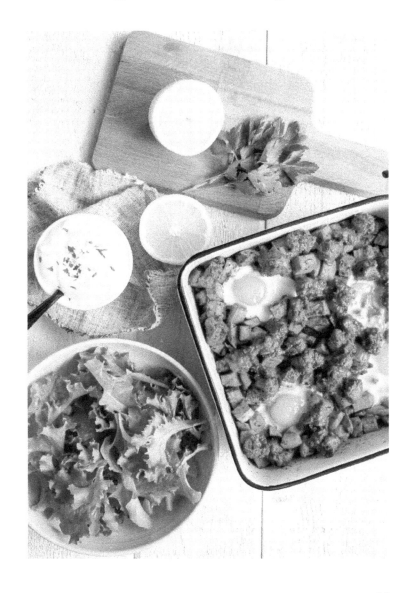

35. Baked Sweet Potato Hash

(Ready in about: 60 minutes | Serving: 4 | Difficulty: Medium)

Nutrition per serving: Kcal 288 | Fat 10 g | Net Carb 10 g | Protein 21 g

Ingredients

- 2 cloves of minced garlic

- 2 tablespoons of olive oil

- Salt and black pepper, to taste

- 1/2 cup of oyster mushrooms

- 1 pound of unpeeled sweet potatoes, cut into cubes

- 1/2 diced red onion

- 2 tablespoons of thyme leaves

- 1/4 cup of goat cheese

- 1 teaspoon of smoked paprika

- Black pepper, to taste

- Chopped herbs

- 5 whole eggs

Instructions

1. Preheat the Traeger to high with a cast-iron skillet.

2. Add oil to skillet with mushrooms, sweet potatoes, salt, and onion. Mix and bake for 20 minutes. Stir once.

3. Add in 1/2 tsp. of paprika, thyme leaves, black pepper, 1 clove of minced garlic. Cook with grill's lid closed. Cook for 10 minutes or until potatoes become browned and onion is tender.

4. Make space for 5 eggs and crack eggs in these spots — Cook for 10 minutes.

5. Serve with cheese, paprika, herbs.

36. Roasted Onion Bacon Salad

(Ready in about: 2 hours & 15 minutes | Serving: 6 | Difficulty: Medium)

Nutrition per serving: Kcal 234 | Fat 8 g | Net Carb 6 g | Protein 20 g

Ingredients

- 1/2 cup of olive oil

- 10 ounce of cherry tomatoes

- 4 yellow onion

- 2 tablespoons red wine vinegar

- 6 slices of bacon

- 2 cups lettuce

- Salt and pepper, to taste

- 1 cucumber

Instructions

1. Preheat the Traeger to 180 °F; use super smoke if possible.

2. Place onions on the grill, cook for 1/2 an hour, and then individually wrap each in foil and place back on the grill.

3. Switch the grill's temperature to 350 °F. Cook onions for 1 hour, take off the grill, and let them cool down.

4. Put bacon on the grill and cook for 30-35 minutes. Take off the grill and crumble.

5. Chop up the roasted onions.

6. In a bowl, mix red wine vinegar, olive oil, salt, and pepper. Whisk well.

7. In a bowl, add tomatoes, lettuce, roasted onions, bacon, cucumber, pour over vinegar mix.

8. Mix well and serve.

37. Veggie Sandwich

(Ready in about: 60 minutes | Serving: 4 | Difficulty: Medium)

Nutrition per serving: Kcal 213 | Fat 9 g | Net Carb 15 g | Protein 19 g

Ingredients

- 4 buns

- 1 small zucchini, eggplant, yellow squash each cut into strips

- 1 and 1/2 cups of chickpeas

- 1 tablespoon garlic minced

- 1/3 cup of tahini

- 1 teaspoon of kosher salt

- 4 tablespoons of lemon juice

- 1/2 cup of ricotta cheese

- 2 tablespoons of olive oil

- 2 Portobello mushroom

- Salt and pepper, to taste

Instructions

1. Preheat the Traeger to 180 °F.

2. Add chickpeas to a baking sheet, bake for 15-20 minutes.

3. In a food processor, add baked chickpeas, tahini, 4 tablespoons of lemon juice, minced garlic, and salt. Pulse until combined, do not over mix.

4. Switch the grill's temperature to 400-500 °F.

5. Coat all vegetables in salt, black pepper, lemon juice, olive oil to taste.

6. Place vegetables directly on grill and gill side up mushrooms.

7. Cook 10-15 minutes for vegetables and 20-25 minutes for mushrooms.

8. In a bowl, add ricotta, salt, pepper, ricotta, 1 clove of minced garlic, and lemon juice (as needed), mix well.

9. Slice buns open and serve grilled vegetables with the cheese mix and tahini mix.

38. Baked Corn Pudding

(Ready in about: 40 minutes | Serving: 6 | Difficulty: Medium)

Nutrition per serving: Kcal 312 | Fat 13 g | Net Carb 14 g | Protein 7 g

Ingredients

- 15 kernel corns

- 3 cloves of chopped garlic

- 3 tablespoons of butter

- 1/2 cup of cream cheese

- 1 cup parmesan cheese

- 1/2 cup of breadcrumbs

- 1 tablespoon of kosher salt

- 1 cup of cheddar cheese

- 1/2 tablespoon of black pepper

- 1 tablespoon of rosemary, chopped

- 1/2 cup of parmesan cheese

- 1 tablespoon of thyme, minced

Instructions

1. Preheat the Traeger to 350 °F.

2. In a pan, add butter and garlic cook for 3-4 minutes. Add all cheese (except for parmesan), corn, cream cheese, salt, pepper.

3. Cook until cheese is melted and transfer to a baking dish.

4. In another bowl, add parmesan cheese, herbs, and bread crumbs.

5. Spread the herbs mix over the corn mix.

6. Bake for 25 minutes.

7. Serve right away.

39. Peach Salsa

(Ready in about: 30 minutes | Serving: 6 | Difficulty: Medium)

Nutrition per serving: Kcal 198 | Fat 8.8 g | Net Carb 2 g | Protein 7 g

Ingredients

- 4 tablespoons of olive oil

- 2 cloves of minced garlic

- 4 peaches, cut into halves

- 4 tomatoes

- 1 diced jalapeno

- Salt, to taste

- 1 Bunch of cilantro leaves, minced

- Juice from 2 limes

Instructions

1. Preheat the Traeger to 500 °F.

2. Mix 2 tablespoons of olive oil and salt into the cut side of the peaches. Place on grill and cook for 20 minutes, until marks appear.

3. Dice the cooled down peaches. In a bowl, add all other ingredients with diced peaches.

4. Serve as a dip.

Chapter 8: Traeger Grill Bonus

Recipes

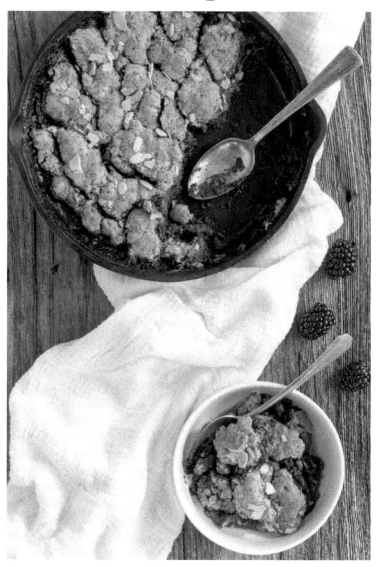

40. Cast Iron Berry Cobbler

(Ready in about: 50 minutes | Serving: 6 | Difficulty: Medium)

Nutrition per serving: Kcal 345 | Fat 25 g | Net Carbs 21 g | Protein 15 g

Ingredients

- 1/2 cup of butter

- 4 cup of berries

- 1/3 cup of orange juice

- 4 tablespoons + 1/2 cup of sugar:

- 2/3 cup of flour

- 1 pinch of salt

- 3/4 teaspoon of baking powder

Instructions

1. Preheat the Traeger to 350 °F with the lid closed for 15 minutes.

2. In a small cast iron pan, mix orange juice, 4 tablespoons of sugar with berries.

3. In a bowl, mix flour, salt, and baking powder.

4. In a bowl, cream the sugar and butter. Add vanilla extract and egg. Fold with flour mix.

5. Spread batter on berries and sprinkle raw sugar.

6. Bake for 35-45 minutes. Serve with cream.

41. Smoked Kentucky Mule

(Ready in about: 10 minutes | Serving: 1 | Difficulty: Easy)

Nutrition per serving: Kcal 55 | Fat 1 g | Net Carbs 0 g | Protein 1 g

Ingredients

- 1/2 ounce of simple smoked syrup
- 2 ounce of high west whiskey
- 4 ounce of ginger beer
- 1 sprig of fresh mint
- 1/2 an ounce of lime juice
- 1 wedge of lime

Instructions

1. In a glass, mix lime juice, ice, whiskey, and simple syrup.

2. Add ginger beer. Mix and serve with mint and line wedge.

42. Smoked Cocktail

(Ready in about: 50 minutes | Serving: 1 | Difficulty: Easy)

Nutrition per serving: Kcal 72 | Fat 1 g | Net Carbs 0 g | Protein 2 g

Ingredients

- 1 and a half-ounce of dry Vermouth

- 1 Jar of soaked cocktail onions

- 1 and a half-ounce of Vodka

Instructions

1. Preheat the Traeger to 180 °F.

2. In a sheet pan, add a jar of cocktail onion. For 45 minutes, smoke it. Take off the grill and set it aside.

3. In a glass, add 1 teaspoon of smoked onions, vodka, dry vermouth. Mix and strain in a glass.

4. Serve with onion on skewers.

43. Smoked Hot Toddy

(Ready in about: 40 minutes | Serving: 1 | Difficulty: Easy)

Nutrition per serving: Kcal 61 | Fat 0 g | Net Carbs 1 g | Protein 1 g

Ingredients

- 1 slice of lemon

- 1 of mint, peach, green tea bag each

- 1 stick of cinnamon

- 1 cup of lemonade

- 1/2 cup of high west double rye

Instructions

1. Preheat the Traeger to 500 °F, with the lid, closed.

2. In a baking dish, add lemonade and put it on the grill. Cook for 20-30 minutes, until internal temperature reaches 200 °F

3. Pour smoked lemonade into a glass. Add all tea bags in lemonade for 2-4 minutes, take them out, and add whiskey.

4. Serve with a cinnamon stick and lemon slice.

44. Garden Gimlet Cocktail

(Ready in about: 50 minutes | Serving: 1 | Difficulty: Easy)

Nutrition per serving: Kcal 56 | Fat 0.9 g | Net Carbs 2 g | Protein 3 g

Ingredients

- 1-and-a-half-ounce Vodka

- 1 cup of honey

- 2 sprig of rosemary

- Zest of 2 lemons

- 2 slices of cucumber

- 1/4 cup of water

- 3/4 ounce of lime juice

Instructions

1. Preheat the Traeger to 180 °F, use super smoke.

2. In a pan, add honey with water, lemon zest, and rosemary.

3. Put the pan on the grill and smoke for 45-60 minutes. Strain and let it cool

4. In a cup, muddle cucumber with lime juice, 1 ounce of rosemary lemon syrup

5. Add ice transfer to a clean glass after straining.

45. Spinach Dip Rollups

(Ready in about: 40 minutes | Serving: 12 | Difficulty: Medium)

Nutrition per serving: Kcal 403 | Fat 35 g | Net Carbs 15 g | Protein 9 g

Ingredients

- 1 roll of crescent dough

- 2 teaspoons of butter

- 6-ounce of baby spinach

- 8-ounce of softened cream cheese

- 1 teaspoon minced garlic

- 2 cups of shredded mozzarella

- 1 cup of mayo

- 1 cup of sour cream

- 1/4 teaspoon of black pepper

- 1 cup of shredded parmesan

- 1/2 teaspoon of salt

Instructions

1. Sauté garlic in butter for 10 seconds, add baby spinach, cook for 2 minutes.

2. In a bowl, mix sour cream, mayo, cream cheese, salt, and pepper.

3. Add in the wilted spinach mix.

4. Add in cheeses, save 1/2 of a cup for later.

5. Roll the crescent dough; use flour so it will not become sticky.

6. Add in the spinach filling and roll the dough.

7. Place on a baking sheet. Top with cheese and bake for 20 to 25 minutes, at 325 °F in Traeger.

8. Slice into single servings and serve.

46. Gin & Tonic

(Ready in about: 55 minutes | Serving: 1 | Difficulty: Easy)

Nutrition per serving: Kcal 77 | Fat 1 g | Net Carbs 2 g | Protein 3 g

Ingredients

- 2 tablespoons of granulated sugar

- 1/4 cup of berries

- 1 sprig of fresh mint

- 1 and a half-ounce of gin

- 1/2 cup of tonic water

- 1 orange, cut into slices

Instructions

1. Preheat the Traeger to 180 °F with the lid closed; use super smoke if possible.

2. Place berries on baking pan and place on grill. Let it smoke for 1/2 an hour at 180 °F.

3. Raise the Traeger temperature to 450 °F with the lid closed.

4. Coat orange slices with sugar and put them directly on the grill — Cook for 5 minutes, or till grill marks appear.

5. In a glass, add berries, ice, gin, and fill with tonic water.

6. Serve with fresh thyme and grilled orange.

Chapter 9: Dressings & Sauces

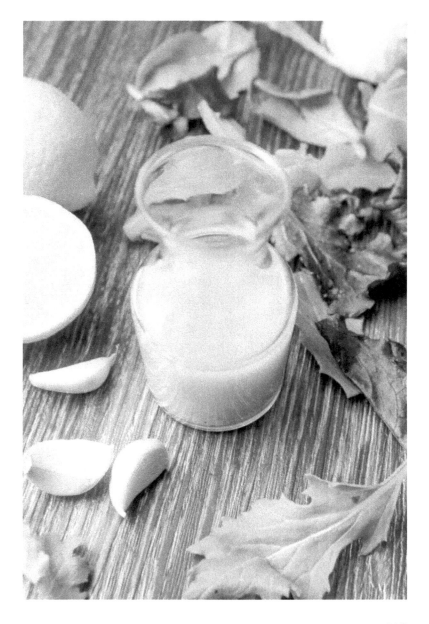

47. Lemon-Garlic Dressing

(Ready in about: 5 minutes | Serving: 8-10 | Difficulty level: easy)

Nutrition per serving: Kcal 81 | Fat 4 g | Protein 6g | Net Carbs 2 g

Ingredients

- 8   cloves of garlic

- Juice of 1 lemon

- 1/8 teaspoon of red pepper flakes

- 1 dash of salt

- 1/4 teaspoon of sea salt

- 1/2 cup of olive oil

Instructions

1. Put all the ingredients in a blender, pulse till combine.

2. Smoke in Traeger for 10 minutes at smoke mode.

3. Let them infuse overnight for better taste.

4. Serve and enjoy.

48. Sweet Potato Caramel

(Ready in about: 15 minutes | Serving: 8-10 | Difficulty level: Easy)

Nutrition per serving: Kcal 150 | Proteins 25 g | Net Carbs 10 g | Fat 8g

Ingredients

- 1 cup of water

- 3 pounds of sweet potatoes, cubed

Instructions

1. Let the oven preheat 425 °F. In a baking dish, put diced potatoes and 1/2 cup of water sealed with foil.

2. Bake for 1 hour, then uncover for 15 minutes. And bake takes out the dish from the oven and uses the 1/2 cup of water to break up some pieces in the dish.

3. Put all the liquids, solids into a cheesecloth-lined strainer. Let it drain and cool in a pan for 1/2 an hour.

4. Squeeze out the juice as much as possible You could end up with a 1-1/2 cup of liquid.

5. Put the sweet potato liquid to a boil in a saucepan, then lower heat for a slow simmer.

6. Let the liquid decrease for almost 20 minutes before it thickens and develops a caramel color.

7. Smoke in Traeger for 20 minutes at smoke mode. Store it in a container in the refrigerator.

49. Creamy Avocado Lime Dressing

(Ready in about: 10 minutes | Serving: 8-10 | Difficulty level: Easy)

Nutrition per serving: Kcal 123 | Fat 12.3g | Net Carbs 4g | Protein 0.8g

Ingredients

- 1/4 cup of olive oil

- 1/4 cup of water

- 1 and 1/2 avocado

- 1/8 teaspoon of pepper

- 1/4 cup of lime juice

- 1/4 cup of cilantro

- 1/4 teaspoon of salt

- 1/8 teaspoons of cumin

- 1/2 teaspoon of crushed garlic

Instruction

1. Put all ingredients in the blender.

2. Pulse till well combined.

3. Smoke in Traeger for 10 minutes at smoke mode.

4. Store or serve right away.

50.   Ranch Coconut Milk Dressing

(Ready in about: 10 minutes | Serving: 8-10 | Difficulty level: Easy)

Nutrition per serving: Kcal 232 | Proteins 25 g | Carbs 15 g | Fat 10g

Ingredients

- 1 can of full-fat coconut milk

- 3 tablespoons of chives

- 1 tablespoon of dill

- 1 and 1/2 tablespoons of basil

- 2 tablespoons of apple cider vinegar

- 2 tablespoons of chopped shallots

- 1 clove of chopped garlic

- 1 teaspoon of sea salt

- Black pepper

- 1 and 1/2 tablespoons of parsley

Instructions

1. Put the coconut cream in a bowl, leave the coconut water behind.

2. Add 4 tablespoons of coconut water to coconut cream, mix until creamy.

3. Add Garlic, shallots, apple cider vinegar, parsley, chives, dill basil, salt, and black pepper. Mix it and at least left in the fridge for 1/2 an hour for flavoring-infusing.

4. Smoke in Traeger for 10 minutes at smoke mode.

5. Enjoy this sauce over favorite foods.

Conclusion

Pellet grills are not a new invention as they have been around for more than three decades, however in recent years they have made a resurgence and improved their functionalities. They can function as a grill or as a smoker, or even combine both functions and include others.

In the case of the Traeger Grill and Smoker, it is a pellet grill that has Trager's 6-in-1 functionality with which you can barbecue, grill, braise, smoke, roast and bake, with the advantage of achieving effective flavors and similar results every time you cook.

All these functionalities will allow you to cook effectively and in the best way, from the simplest to the most complicated recipes. According to the type of food and the recipe instructions, you can cook on high heat, or you can cook on low and slow, which is really the perfect middle ground. Regardless of the cooking method, all your recipes will have a spectacular flavor that will make you look like a grilling pro.

CPSIA information can be obtained
at www.ICGtesting.com
Printed in the USA
BVHW070856150321
602550BV00010B/1190